High Styles

To purchase this book for resale, as a fundraising project or in a retail outlet, contact iUniverse toll free at 1-877-288-4737 or on the web at <www.iuniverse.com>.

High Styles

Stories from a World Class Hairdresser

by Buddy Walton
with Connie McIntyre

iUniverse, Inc.
New York Lincoln Shanghai

High Styles
Stories from a World Class Hairdresser

iUniverse, Inc.

For information address:
iUniverse, Inc.
2021 Pine Lake Road, Suite 100
Lincoln, NE 68512
www.iuniverse.com

Front Cover Photo: World renowned hairdresser Buddy Walton and his model, Luci, add some finishing touches at the 1964 World Championships of Hairdressing in Paris.

ISBN: 0-595-31875-4

Printed in the United States of America

Dedicated to my devoted and skilled receptionist
Marie Weisser
and to my dear friend and mentor
Miss Edna Emme
president of Godefroy Cosmetics
manufacturer of TRESemmé hair products

High Styles

Contents

Introduction

For as long as I can remember, I have loved working with hair. That's just how I am. I was a licensed cosmetologist for more than fifty-five years, starting in the business when a haircut cost three dollars and a style cost five. I waited on people from all walks of life—people from my small boyhood town of Mineral Point, near Potosi, Missouri; people in St. Louis, Missouri high society; and political figures, movie stars, and celebrities from around the world. I waited on the First Ladies of St. Louis, the First Ladies of Missouri, and the First Ladies of the United States. I waited on the Queen of Sweden and Countess Torniski of Poland. I waited on Joan Crawford, Sophie Tucker, Abigail van Buren, and so many others.

I headed three salons in St. Louis and four in Florida. Twenty-three times, I represented the National Hairdresser and Cosmetologist Association (NHCA) at various European events. I served as an NHCA Team Advisor in Japan and took part in the first American hairdressing demonstration in Russia. I was honored to have my name on many trophies, such as Buddy Walton's Roving Cup, and to serve as a judge at national and international events.

Looking back, I'm surprised. Why should all this happen to me, a little old guy from a little town in Missouri?

Roots

Making Waves

I've had a marvelous life. Now I've reached an age where people ask me how old I am. When they do, I tell them that I have a twin brother. They think I'm making it up, but I do have a twin brother. Then I tell them that I am ten years younger than he is. Let me just say that in the first half of the 1900s, in my small Missouri hometown, male hairstylists were unheard of. Hairdressing was considered a female profession. But I enjoyed creating hairstyles, even as a young boy.

My twin brother, Rusty, and I were the youngest of five brothers; I had good, smart brothers. When my older brothers and my parents played cards, which they did often, my dad would always take the host chair, the one with arms. I was my father's favorite. I'd sit on his shoulders, with my feet on the arms of the chair. I'd have a glass of water nearby, and I'd wave his hair while he played cards. My dad would let me do anything.

Rusty and I never looked much alike, and we certainly never shared many interests. My mother would take Rusty to boxing class and me to dancing school. Rusty was fixing flat tires and broken motors while I was putting makeup on the girl next door. When I was in elementary school, the tunic dress was very smart—straight, no waist, and short, just below the knees. I would take my mother's tunic dresses, while she was at work, and dress up all the boys my age and put makeup on them and have a show. I ruined many of her dresses by getting lipstick on them. I was different than the rest of them, I will admit. When Rusty and I reached driving age, he was allowed to drive anywhere he wanted, but my parents didn't trust me—I wasn't mechanically inclined. I usually had the lead in the school play and things like that, activities where I wouldn't get dirty.

My mother taught school, and my father was postmaster. They had five sons to raise and to educate—how did they do it? They were just good people. We had a good life. When I was quite a young boy, Harry Truman was senator. He and my father were both active Masons, a tradition my brothers and I have continued. My mother would often say to my twin brother and me, "You babies will have to eat early because the Senator is coming to town and your father and older brother are going with him to campaign." Little did I know at the time that someday Senator Truman would be our president, and that Mrs. Truman and their daughter, Margaret, would come to my salon.

By the time I was fifteen years old, I knew I had a flair for hairdressing. Still, I followed in my older brothers' footsteps after I finished high school and attended Warrensburg Teacher's College. Before the end of the first year, I knew I didn't want to go back. I didn't like it. In spite of negative pressure from my brothers, I wanted to be a hairdresser. My mother and father consented. If that was what I wanted to do, I could do it. My father took me to Moler College in downtown St. Louis, Missouri. Every day for two weeks, my father accompanied me from my uncle's home, to the streetcar, and on to the school. At the end of the day, he was waiting outside the school to accompany me on the return trip. I was such a baby, afraid of the big city, and he was so patient.

Even early in my training, people liked my work. They came into the school salon, asking for me to do their hair. When I graduated, Mr. Pruitt, the top instructor, wrote in my textbook, "The greatest male hairdresser I have ever taught cosmetology."

I was a dreamer then, and I still am. I can remember standing in a huge window of Moler College in downtown St. Louis, watching drivers of beautiful cars pass by on the street below, and wishing that someday it could be me. My wish came true, but I did more than succeed. I did what I wanted to do, what I had dreamed of doing my whole life. I did what I loved.

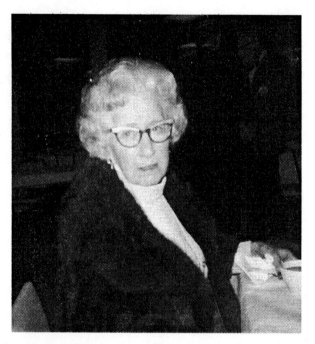

Mother Walton lived to be one hundred years old. She was ninety-eight when this photo was taken.

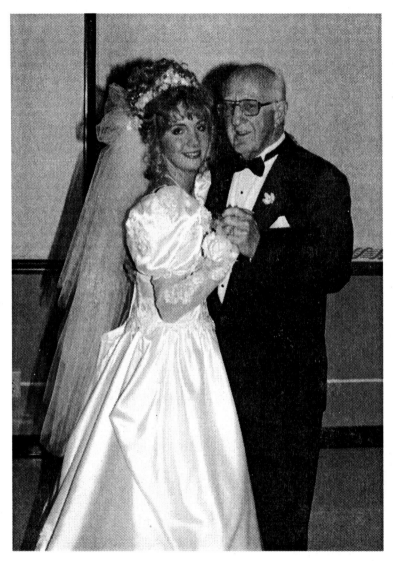

My twin brother, Rusty, dances with the bride, his granddaughter Bry. Bry was named after one of my best friends and favorite clients, Mrs. Erwin Bry.

Getting Set

My first hairdresser job was with Marian Miles and Hatti Cordia Coleman in Potosi, my hometown. My mother—as mothers are—was afraid that I would stay home and not amount to anything. She got me a job away from home, at a shop in Festus, Missouri, at fifteen dollars a week. She also got me a place to live in the Methodist minister's home. I can see myself going to work early in the morning, walking down the railroad track because I couldn't afford a car.

A cousin of mine was a hairdresser in downtown St. Louis, at the De Soto Hotel. She wanted to take a vacation and asked me to work for her while she was gone. It was quite a change for me, from quiet Festus, Missouri to busy downtown St. Louis. My cousin never came back to her job, so I stayed on. I was young and inexperienced, but I had customers who requested me, such as Mrs. Simon, whose husband was the manager of the De Soto and Claridge hotels, and who remained my customer for years.

I had been there for a few months when George Lutkewette, a popular hair supply salesman, took an interest in me. After watching me work, he asked me if I would consider moving to a bigger salon. I said, "George, what place are you thinking of?" And he told me about an elegant residential hotel in the Central West End, the Congress Hotel. George called the hotel, and the owners, Irene and Gay, were interested, so I made the switch. After a couple of successful years at the Congress, George again helped me move up, to a position in the popular Chase Hotel. "The Chase is the Place." It was true at that time, as it is now.

When I had been at the Chase a couple of years, I received an offer from Eugene Gossoux, owner of the Park Plaza Beauty Salon. Two fellow employees and most of my customers followed me when I made the move. Soon afterward, the two hotels combined to become the Chase Park Plaza Hotel.

After a time, an exclusive apartment building, the Montclair, was built just a few blocks from the Chase Park Plaza, on South Kingshighway. I was contacted about opening a salon there. I was excited and frightened at the prospect of going out on my own, but with some financial assistance from my parents, I did so. I didn't tell Mr. Gossoux or Mr. and Mrs. Sam Koplar, owners of the Chase Park Plaza, but word of my plans got around. One day, Mr. Gossoux said to me, "Buddy, I hate to do this, but I think that today will be your last day." My salon wasn't quite ready, so for a few weeks I worked out of a shop on De Balivere, owned by my friend Erwin Katzman. Through it all, my clients, including some of the most well-known people in St. Louis, stayed with me, as did Marie, the receptionist; Florence Sofois, another top stylist who became half owner of the Montclair Salon; and a number of other staff people.

I was thrilled to own my own shop! United States Treasurer Amy Priest had been a customer of mine at the Chase Park Plaza. Remembering her suggestion, I kept the first dollar I made at the Montclair and at every shop I opened from then on.

I served a number of interesting clients at my Montclair salon, such as Princess Tarnoski of Poland. She and her cousin, who was also a Polish princess, were in exile in St. Louis, having escaped Poland in anticipation of a German invasion. They were very fine clients. I often saw them attend the opera and the ballet.

Mrs. Elizabeth Cavenaugh, who lived in the building, was another of my memorable Montclair customers. She loved diamonds. She had fifty-eight diamonds in her black-rimmed glasses, across the front and along the earpieces. Most were one-carat; a couple were four-carat. She also had diamond studs around the tops of her ears to continue the lines, which each ended, of course, with a diamond earring that dangled brightly. Mrs. Cavenaugh carried on the theme with diamond rings on her hands, diamond bracelets, diamond necklaces, and a diamond watch. She'd smile at you and say, "I like diamonds." She was robbed several times because she rode the bus downtown to do her shopping and told people on the bus that those were *diamonds* in her glasses.

Mrs. Cavenaugh had her hair styled and shampooed every other week. We often found parrot feathers in her hair, from her pet parrot, which she loved. We enjoyed having Mrs. Cavenaugh as a client. She eventually sold her midtown St. Louis property at Grand and Olive for development, and she did quite well for herself.

Mrs. Koplar, of the Chase Park Plaza, called me after I had been at the Montclair for almost two years. I was surprised to hear from her and shocked by what she had to say. "I'm going to ask you a question," she said. "How would you like to come home?"

I didn't know what she meant.

"How would you like to come back to the Chase Park Plaza?" she asked.

It was quite a compliment, but I didn't know what to say. Though my salon at the Montclair had been successful, it wasn't quite paid for.

"Oh, don't worry about the money," she said. "If you want to come back, we'll give it to you. We know what you can do with the space."

It was a very happy day. I did go back to the Chase Park Plaza and it was good to be home. If anyone had told me then how fantastic the next thirty-five years would be, if they had even hinted at the friends I would make, the people I would meet, and the awards I would earn while working in my Chase Park Plaza salon, I would not have believed it. I can hardly believe it now.

The Elite Set

I enjoyed working in my salon in the Chase Park Plaza Hotel for thirty-five years, waiting on the elite of St. Louis and the world. People liked me and liked how I did hair. They came back and brought their friends, until the salon grew from three or four hairdressers to nearly forty employees—hairdressers, manicurists, a masseuse, and the world's most wonderful receptionist, Marie Weisser. The shop was not only professional, it was fun. We were often interrupted by celebrities coming in to say hello—Bob Hope, Phyllis Diller, Margo Fontaine, and so many others.

Mr. and Mrs. Koplar, and later, their son Harold, were so good to me and good to work with. Of course, they expected you to produce. I was once walking through the lower level of the hotel with Mr. Sam Koplar. A hotel employee was on the floor, asleep. When his fellow employee saw us coming, he ran up to the man who was sleeping, saying, "Wake up! Wake up! Here comes the boss!"

Mr. Koplar said, "Oh, don't wake him up. He has a job until you wake him up."

One day when Mrs. Koplar was in my salon, she told me a surprising story. She said to me, "Buddy, see the lady over there? I have to tell you about her. She is very wealthy, but she once did something quite unexpected—she tried to take my sheets!

"When I owned the Branson Hotel, she had an apartment with us. Then she decided to move to the new Montclair apartments on Kingshighway. One of my housemen discovered that she was keeping hotel sheets and pillowcases in a dresser drawer to move with her. But I fooled her. We replaced the sheets she was stealing with old, torn, cut-up sheets that we laundered, pressed, and folded. I hope she was very shocked when she got to the Montclair and found she had to buy new sheets!"

My Favorite Ladies

Many wealthy ladies came to my Chase Park Plaza salon. Most were very generous to me, some beyond belief, and many became friends as well as clients. Mrs. Erwin Bry was especially generous; the best gift she gave me was friendship.

Mrs. Bry had her hair done several times a week, sometimes on Sundays. She was so generous to me that I could never say *no* to her. She wore her hair short and tossed, and with color. It was a natural look, very fashionable.

In later years, after Mr. Bry's death, my friendship with Mrs. Bry grew. I had dinner with her in her apartment nearly every Wednesday. The delicious meals were prepared by Florence, Mrs. Bry's excellent cook and personal assistant, and served by Florence or the butler. We socialized together at various St. Louis country clubs—I'm sure we were the talk of the city. Several times we flew to Cleveland, where we were entertained by her brother and sister-in-law. Mrs. Bry's maiden name was Richman; her family owned Richman Brothers Clothing Company, which originated in Cleveland. Also while we were in Cleveland, we were entertained by executives of the May Company, which had quite a representation there.

Whenever Mrs. Bry and I traveled together, which was often, I kept her hair looking its best each day. We took yearly trips to

Florida, as well as several shopping trips to New York City. One time, we went to Europe. Another time, we took a cruise to South America. At each stop on the cruise, we had a chauffeured limousine to take us anywhere we wanted to go.

During most of my years at the Chase Park Plaza, I lived in a beautiful home on Lindell Boulevard. On departure day, Mrs. Bry's chauffeured limousine would pick me up. Behind her limousine, Vera, my longtime maid, drove my car with our luggage. We often had a police escort to the airport, where we never had to wait in line.

I have wondered why Mrs. Bry was so kind to me. In addition to her friendship, she gave me thousands of dollars over a period of years and also left me a sizable sum in her will. She was undoubtedly the finest lady I have ever met.

Mrs. Bry was a very good friend of another favorite customer of mine, the lovely Mrs. Millard Waldheim. Mrs. Waldheim's father was Morton May, of the May Company and Famous Barr. Her husband, Millard, was also a friend of mine. He reportedly left $46 million to Jewish Hospital when he died.

In the early years, Mrs. Waldheim wore her hair in a short pageboy. Later, she switched to a smart, shorter cut, with the latest innovation—highlighting. I was one of the first in St. Louis to offer my customers highlighting.

The Waldheims gave wonderful parties in the Khorassan Room at the Chase Park Plaza Hotel or at their Kentucky home, where they were known for their beautiful New Year's parties. Their guest lists generally included several hundred of their best friends from all over the country. I was lucky to be included. Mrs. Waldheim overheard a relative at one of her parties say, "Oh,

Lord. There's Buddy Walton. Don't they ever give a party without him?"

And Mrs. Waldheim said to her, "Yes, Buddy is always invited. Buddy's invited because he's a friend. You're invited because you're a relative."

Guests were treated like royalty at a Waldheim party. At the Chase Park Plaza, the parties were usually black tie dinners. Music during and after dinner was provided by the best local talent, like Jack Denett, or the Waldheims flew in big-name orchestra leaders, such as Guy Lombardo. Dancing was popular then, and I loved to dance for hours. One of my favorite dancing partners was Thelma Propstein Katz, whose mother was a Koplar.

I'll never forget the first time I attended a party at the Waldheims' Kentucky home. They had flown me there on their private plane, as they did on several occasions. Among the guests were some other very notable St. Louis people, such as Mrs. Ben Loeb, Mr. and Mrs. Henry Stern, Mrs. Jack Edlin, and many others who happened to be clients of mine. I woke up early and decided to see the house by myself. It was a huge house. As I went downstairs, I saw Mrs. Waldheim sitting alone at an enormous table, waiting for her guests to come for breakfast. She said, "Buddy, I'm so glad to see you. Come in and be seated." She was at the extreme right end of one side of the long table. Instead of asking where I should be seated, I went to the head of the table to sit down next to her. She said, "Oh, Buddy, don't sit at the head. Millard will sit there."

I should have known. There was a lot I had to learn. But the home and grounds were beautiful. Some nights I stayed up late to see a horse foal. And I went to horse races with them. I didn't know about races. One time I said, "Oh, I have the winning ticket!

Here it is!" But then I dropped it, and it fell to the ground among hundreds and hundreds of tickets that all looked the same. I thought, "Oh, Lord. How will I find my ticket?" But Mrs. Waldheim helped me look for it; she was down on her hands and knees with me.

The Waldheims were awfully good to me. For many years, I received quite a sizable check at Christmas and on other occasions, amounting to thousands of dollars. On my fiftieth birthday, Mrs. Waldheim and Mrs. Gordon Scherck, another favorite client, gave me a large party at Westwood Country Club, and many prominent St. Louis people were there.

Many times, I flew to New York City with Mrs. Waldheim, maybe to select a wig or just to shop. We always stayed at the famous Pierre Hotel. Her sister-in-law Helen Platt lived there, and we always had her chauffeur at our disposal. Mrs. Waldheim and I often had dinner together in St. Louis, and frequently she also invited my mother. I was having dinner with Mrs. Waldheim the evening that she had her stroke. That was twenty years ago. I still am with her every Thursday as she has her hair done by Steve Smith, who was once a stylist in my salon.

Mr. and Mrs. Shenker often invited me to their parties, too. Mrs. Shenker, the Koplars' daughter, was a judge and quite a lady. She and her husband, Morris, one of the top criminal lawyers in the United States, also owned the Dunes Hotel in Las Vegas. The Shenkers entertained ambassadors and other world figures at the Chase Park Plaza, and I was very flattered, on more than one occasion, to be invited. As I did Mrs. Shenker's hair prior to one such event, I placed clips in the sides of her hair to hold it very close, per her usual request. I always said to her, "Don't forget to take these clips out of your hair."

And she always said, "Put them in. I won't forget."

As we were in line, shaking hands with the dignitaries, I looked up and saw the clips in Mrs. Shenker's hair. I very nonchalantly took them out and put them in my pocket.

Not every invitation was welcome. Mr. and Mrs. Huntsinger lived a few doors from me on Lindell Boulevard. Mr. Huntsinger was a prominent professor at Washington University. Mrs. Huntsinger was giving a small brunch, and I was invited. Some very well-known people were on the guest list: Mr. and Mrs. Edward Grossman, world travelers from St. Louis; Lord and Lady Peter and Do Jean Smithers of London; Lady Do Jean's mother, Mrs. Louella Sayman, whose husband was very successful with Sayman Soap; and a leading archaeologist of Greece and his wife.

I was uncomfortable at the thought of attending a small brunch with such distinguished people whom I didn't know. I gave the excuse that my mother would be in town, and I had to spend the day with her. Mrs. Huntsinger said, "Buddy, you are so good around ladies, and my husband isn't. I wish you could be there to help me entertain." I repeated this to several of my well-to-do clients in the salon, and they all insisted that I attend. I called Mrs. Huntsinger back and told her that my plans had changed; I could accept her invitation after all.

As I approached the house on the day of the luncheon, I saw that it was surrounded by limousines. My nervousness increased. When we moved toward the brunch table, Mrs. Sayman said, "Buddy, you sit by me."

While brunch was being served, the guests took turns introducing themselves. I kept wondering to myself, "How am I going to introduce myself? 'Buddy the hairdresser?'"

When it was my turn, Mrs. Sayman looked at her daughter, Do Jean, and said, "Do Jean, you do know Buddy Walton, don't you? He is one of the foremost hairdressers in the United States—in fact, in the world."

I felt so relieved. Then Mrs. Betty Grossman asked about Lady Do Jean's daughter, Sarah.

"Oh, Betty," Lady Do Jean said. "You haven't read the newspapers lately. Sarah is in Sarasota learning to be a trapeze artist."

I felt even better.

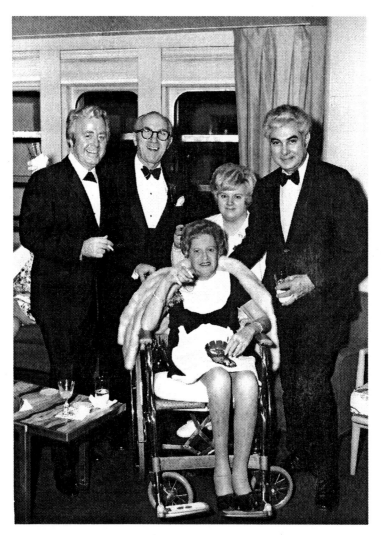

We stopped for a photo while on our South American cruise.
That's Mr. Buddy (me) on the left, Mrs. Bry in the center, and
my friend Sam Micotto on the right. Samie Cohen and Mrs.
Bry's nurse, Carol Ann, stand behind.

Photo by Grace Line Publicity Department, New York City

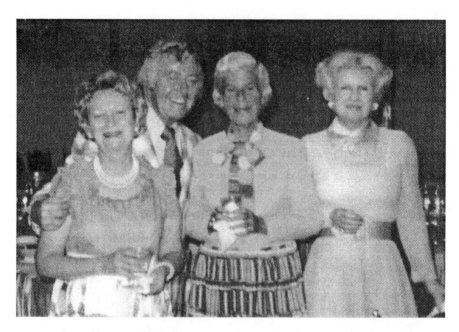

My fiftieth birthday party at Westwood Country Club included
many prominent people of St. Louis. Left to right: Mrs.
Millard Waldheim, Mrs. Gordon Scherck, and Mrs. Lewis
Bettman. Mrs. Scherck often told me that I could do her hair
better with one hand than any other hairdresser in St. Louis
could with two hands.

Society Snips

Years ago, hairstyling was very different than it is now. Ladies would sometimes come in to get their hair washed and styled two or three times a week. Some had their hair combed every day. I got to know many of my customers very well. One of my very favorite ladies was Mrs. Don Lambert, a popular society lady. Mrs. Lambert was very particular. She would buy six or eight dresses from Saks Fifth Avenue or Montaldo's and have them delivered to her home on Westmoreland Place, across the street from my salon. After I finished work, I was expected to go by her house and help her decide which dresses she should keep.

Mrs. Lambert liked her hair in a tight curl and attempted to schedule a new permanent wave more often than was advisable. Perms were expensive; even then, they were fifty dollars. Once when I refused to give her a perm because her hair was not yet ready for it, she had the work done at a neighboring salon. The next day, she was back in my salon, asking for my help. I did what I could to get her hair back in condition. She was one of my favorite ladies.

Mr. and Mrs. Wooster Lambert, of the pharmaceutical business that has become Warner Lambert Consumer Health Care, were among the supporters of Lindbergh's famous flight. They lived at the Park Plaza, and Mrs. Lambert was another of my favorite ladies, though she demanded certain things that were so unusual. When she had an appointment, the styling chair, the shampoo chair, the shampoo basin, the top of the dresser—everything had to be wiped off with disinfectant soap. She did not like to touch anything that other people had touched. She brought her own hair rollers, her own clips, her own hair net—everything that would touch her. (We used hair nets because the older dryers blew the hair.) We both laughed one day when I said to her, "Mrs. Lambert, you're a very nice lady. I wouldn't take a million dollars for you, but you know, I wouldn't give a nickel for another one like you."

One of my very favorite customers—there were so may favorites— was Mrs. Trudy Busch, Gussie Busch's wife. When she was in town, she was in the salon every week. We had dinner together many times. When she was getting divorced, she'd call me and say, "You wanna go here? You wanna go there?"

Of course, not every customer became a friend. I went to one lady's apartment, in a condo on Hanley Road in nearby Clayton, to cut her hair. I knocked on her door and she said to me, after I came in, "Buddy, do me a favor."

And I said, "I certainly will, if I can."

She said, "Next time, knock on the kitchen door, will you?"

I said, "No, I won't." I said, "I've been invited to the homes of Mrs. Bry, Mrs. Waldheim, Mrs. Busch, Mrs. Lambert…They have never told me not to come in the front entrance. Next week you can get someone else to do your hair." She apologized then, but I told her I would not be back. A very nice woman I know moved into this same lady's apartment building and suggested they have lunch together sometime. The lady's response was, "My time is filled." But those people are fun to talk about.

One of my most extraordinary customers was Mrs. Carolyn Burford. Her maiden name was Skelly, of Skelly Oil. I was once told how Mrs. Burford and her daughter had a terrible argument that resulted in them cutting up their mink coats! I used to go to Mrs. Burford's home, on Portland Place, to do her hair. A secretary worked at a desk on the second floor of her home, next to a ticker tape machine reporting New York Stock Exchange activity. That was quite a sight. Mrs. Burford later purchased the Busch home on Lindbergh, a huge home with a large acreage. She was often robbed—over a period of years, she experienced jewelry thefts totaling around twenty million dollars—but she refused to buy insurance. She preferred to pick up the phone and order new jewels. I read somewhere that Mrs. Burford's income was $300,000 a day, but she served peanut butter and jelly sandwiches at a black tie dinner. I understand that when Mrs. Burford died, she left $17 million, and her property was sold to a subdivision developer for another $17 million. She also left a debt of $250 to my salon. Never paid it. I liked her anyway.

A surprising and unusual friendship developed between me and a striking young woman who came into my salon. We enjoyed talking while I did her hair, and she called me later. She wanted to know if I had a friend who could take her and her friend out to dinner. My friend Sam and I went out to dinner with Bobbie and her friend, Cecilia. We all became friends. They spent a lot of time in my St. Louis home, and Sam and I visited them in California. We stayed in a nearby hotel but enjoyed all the lavishness of their beautiful Santa Monica home, including a steam-heated pool and every other luxury you can imagine, plus a chauffeur, who was available to us at all times.

Over time, we discovered that Bobbie's extravagant lifestyle was a "gift" from Andy Norman, husband of Merle Norman, of Merle Norman Cosmetics. We also learned that Bobbie and Cecilia were more than just friends. Andy Norman thought they were sisters and supported them both. He would buy two sets of every gift: a diamond bracelet, necklace, and earrings for each of them; a sapphire ring, earrings, and necklace for each; minks for both of them. Later, when Andy Norman was suffering from cancer and Bobbie was making numerous trips to the hospital to be with him, she fell in love with the chauffeur. After Andy Norman's death, Bobbie married the chauffeur. The ceremony took place in Las Vegas. Though I was not able to attend, Sam did. Unfortunately, Bobbie accidentally choked to death at an early age.

Many other interesting people became my customers in my Chase Park Plaza salon. Unforgettable Mrs. Liz Rubin, who was a regular in the salon, was known for her...how should I say it... distinctive parties. At one such event, she declared in a voice every guest could hear, "I'm the only woman in Washington Terrace who has the nerve to have a loud party with all the loose ladies and gay boys under the roof at one time."

Mrs. Mrazek, of the United Van Lines business, became my client by recommendation of a friend. After waiting on her for a year or two, she became a very good, and generous, friend. She told me that she lost and gained weight rapidly, so when she bought a dress that she really liked, she would buy it in three or four sizes and have one of them fitted, as needed. That way, a dress that she liked was always available to wear. She chose very expensive designer dresses.

Mrs. Phillips was always cold. She always wore a coat. One day, one of my boys was giving her a perm, and she refused to take off her coat, as usual. He gave her the perm, and when he was ready to rinse her hair, he found that he had wrapped the fur of her coat's collar in the perm roller. She just laughed and said it was her fault.

Almost anything could happen in my salon—or *almost* happen. We had a phone call one day from a man who lived in Arcadia, Missouri. My receptionist, Marie, called out, "Who's expecting a call from Arcadia, Missouri?" Marie didn't know that the man's wife and his girlfriend were both in the salon. They almost ran into each other as they dashed to the phone! One lady actually threatened to shoot Marie if she booked a "certain lady" for an appointment. That "certain lady" was her husband's girlfriend, and they both came to my shop. We had many occasions like that; we had to be very careful.

My clients sometimes told me stories that I thought were so funny. Society lady Mrs. John Simon, of John Simon Securities, lived in the Park Plaza, and below her lived Mrs. Sam Simon, whose husband manufactured the London Fog raincoat. Mrs. Sam Simon came in for me to do her hair one winter day, and she was very perturbed. She said that Mrs. John Simon, in the apartment above her, had called and said, "Mrs. Simon, I rinsed out my gloves and put them on the terrace to dry, but the wind blew them down to your terrace. Would you have your maid go out and get them and bring them up to me?"

"Buddy," Mrs. Sam Simon said to me, "I thought it was a lot of nerve, and I told her, 'Indeed not.' If she wanted her gloves, she could send *her* maid down to my apartment and let *her* go out and get them. I wasn't going to let *my* maid catch cold."

Many of my customers drove a distance to receive my services. Mrs. Rosalind Goldman owned Goldman Department Store in Festus, Missouri. Mrs. Edward Eversole also drove in from Festus, where her husband served as one of the Jefferson County Circuit Court judges. Mrs. E. H. Sumner came to St. Louis periodically from Stewart, Mississippi. My friend James Viar, a well-known stylist of Memphis, Tennessee, suggested to Mrs. Sumner that she see me if she needed any hair care while in St. Louis. She came in often through the years, for a haircut, perm, or color. Mrs. Sumner gave $50 million to Mississippi schools.

Missouri senator Edward Long's wife and daughter drove in from out-state Missouri the day before an appointment and stayed at the Chase Park Plaza. They spent several hours with me for haircuts, perms, and so on. Senator Long's daughter was married in the Baptist Church on Grand Avenue and Washington Boulevard in St. Louis, with the reception held at the Chase Park Plaza Hotel. I was invited; it was quite an affair. For years, they remained friends of mine.

Mrs. Needles of Belleville was a weekly customer of mine for years. As a hobby, she raised Black Angus cattle. As she was awaiting the birth of a calf that was expected to be especially fine, she told me she planned to name it *Mr. Buddy*. One day, she came in laughing. "I have bad news for you, Mr. Buddy. The prize Angus calf I've been waiting for turned out to be a heifer!"

Mrs. Erwin, known as the wealthiest widow in Illinois, regularly drove down from Quincy, Illinois for highlights and perms. She became a very good friend. She would stay the night, we would have dinner, and she would get her hair done.

No one came as far as Mrs. Groves. Due to his work in the oil business, Mr. and Mrs. Prof Groves, from my hometown of Potosi,

Missouri, moved to South America. Mrs. Groves came back to Missouri at least three times a year, and when she did, she always called me for a haircut and a perm. I was told that when she died, she left several million dollars to the Missouri Botanical Garden.

I will always remember the one-time customer who came to me from Kansas City. I received a long distance emergency phone call from a woman in distress. After applying a highlighting solution, her hairdresser discovered he couldn't remove the highlighting cap. The lightening solution had made her hair swell so much that it could not be pulled back through the tiny holes in the rubber cap. She chartered a plane to St. Louis so that I could help her. I worked with her for several hours, carefully snipping the cap into small pieces, which I removed one by one. Things like that happen.

I had many loyal St. Louis customers, including Mrs. Fuller, of Stix Baer & Fuller; her daughter Carol Fihnn; Mrs. Kay Qually, who planned her vacation time to be in Florida when I was there; and Mrs. David Wohll, of Wohll Shoe Company, who with her husband has contributed so much to Barnes Jewish Hospital and to our city. Longtime client Mrs. Bonnie Kiefer was like a sister to me. She presented me with fabulous gifts and invited me to every party she gave, remaining loyal and good to me for many years in spite of numerous changes in her personal life. Helen Wolff continued to make regular trips to my salon even after her husband became seriously ill. She told me that he never failed to notice when she had "been to see Buddy." Mrs. Bertie Schirmer, mother of my well-known friend Lloyd Schirmer, Chairman of the Board of Directors of the Smithsonian Institute, was my client forever— until she was 101 years old. In fact, she drove herself to her appointments until she was 100. I still call her and send flowers on special occasions.

My clients were loyal to me, and I was loyal to them. I often visited Mrs. Samuels in her hospital room. When Mrs. Bry was in the hospital, I always had dinner with her, delivered by one of St. Louis' top restaurants. The same was true for Mrs. Eva Baskowitz. When I visited Mrs. Baskowitz in her home following a hospital stay, she traditionally had a surprise for me. "Open the vault," she would order. I would swing the framed picture away from the wall on its hinges, revealing her jewelry vault. Then she would tell me the combination so I could open the vault to see whatever piece of jewelry it was that she wanted to show me. She often had a gift for me.

One of my devoted customers stepped in and made a phone call that changed the future of hairdressing as well as the future of my shop. A national union had decided that hair salons should become unionized and chose to start with my salon. A picket line appeared without notice on Kingshighway and Maryland Avenue, in front of the Chase Park Plaza Hotel. My faithful client Liz Rubin called her influential husband, and within fifteen minutes the picketers were gone.

Many of my clients were very generous to me at Christmas and for my birthday, and a number of them have left me in their wills. As a young man, as I started making a little money and wasn't used to it, I wasted my fair share. It was foolish but wonderful. I once flew to New York to buy a dog from Count Pulaski, who raised prize poodles. I bought my first poodle, Cricket, when I shouldn't have because I really didn't have the money for such a purchase. I paid two thousand dollars. Soon, poodles became so popular that I opened what I think was the second dog grooming shop in St. Louis, at the Chase Park Plaza Hotel. I named it the Poodle Palace. My friend Sam, whose sister Marie was my receptionist, owned it for many years.

Thank goodness I met Mrs. Charlotte Cohen, who became my stockbroker and financial advisor. Charlotte gave me much confidence when I was younger. It is easier to be confident when you don't have to worry too much about other things, like money. Charlotte helped me start investing, but had very little to work with at first because I had very little to invest. As years went on, she helped me build up my stock report. Charlotte, whose husband's family owned Central Hardware, was the first woman in the United States to open a full-service brokerage firm, in 1973. Charlotte also made investments for my mother, who lived to be one hundred years old. Many times, my mother and I remarked, "Thank God for Charlotte."

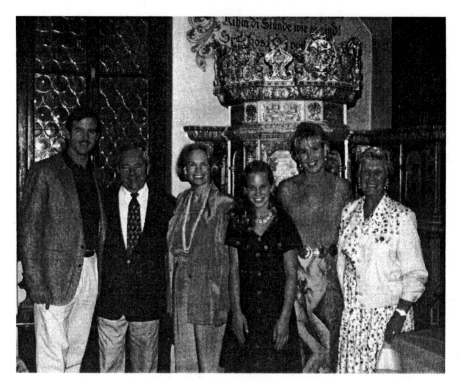

Trudy Busch sent me this photograph when she and Gussie
vacationed with their family in Switzerland. Trudy and I often
went "out on the town" together.

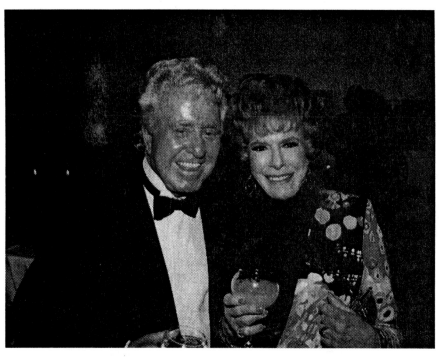

Beautiful Charlotte Cohen is my good friend as well as my
financial adviser.

Heads of State

Through the years, I waited on the wives of many Missouri governors and senators, at times traveling to Jefferson City to do their hair for fundraisers and to release new hairstyles. I've also waited on the wives of St. Louis mayors: Mayor Darst's wife, Mayor Cervantes' wife, and Mayor Tucker's wife. I served Marcella Slay Komorek, Mayor Slay's aunt, for many years. Mayor Slay still sends me a Christmas card every year, and I am proud to support him.

I waited on the mayors' wives often enough that we came to know each other well. When I welcomed Mrs. Cervantes for her appointment one day, I asked, "How are you, Mrs. Cervantes?"

"Fine, but I'm so mad," she said. "I don't know why Jerry Berger dislikes me so."

Mrs. Cervantes explained that the well-known St. Louis gossip columnist had written, "I saw Carmen Cervantes at a party last night with her new face."

Mrs. Tucker was forthright with me, as well. One day when she was in the salon, I said, "Mrs. Tucker, I would like to cut a sample of your hair." She was such a lovely lady.

She was surprised. "Buddy, why do you want that?"

I explained to her that I have collected hair samples from some very important people: Eleanor Roosevelt, Bess Truman, Margaret Truman, Mrs. Nixon...I have collected hair samples from the wives of St. Louis mayors: Mayor Darst's wife, Mayor Cervantes' wife...

"You're not getting *my* hair," she interrupted. "I don't like that lady!"

I've long ago forgotten what the feud was between Mayor Tucker and Mayor Cervantes, but I do remember that one of my stylists gave Mrs. Tucker a perm one day, and I got quite a curl for my collection.

Thanks to my hairdressing career, I also met many national political figures. Eleanor Roosevelt was to make an appearance at a St. Louis luncheon, to autograph a book she had written, and honored me by requesting that I comb her hair. She was such a gracious lady. After Mrs. Roosevelt left, each of the women in my salon told me she felt that as Mrs. Roosevelt spoke, she had looked directly at her. I had felt the same way. Her visit was one of my greatest experiences.

President Truman's wife, Bess, was in town at the same time, as Mrs. Roosevelt's guest, and I had the privilege of combing her hair, too. She had a good cut. Another time, Bess and Margaret Truman visited my salon as they waited to have lunch with Mrs. Charlotte Mandel, in the Gourmet Room of the hotel. Suddenly, I discovered that someone had left my salon's interior door open, and my dogs were missing. Lo and behold, I found all three of my poodles on Margaret's lap, as she sat waiting on the mezzanine.

My mother was very active in Eastern Star, as was President Truman's sister, Mary Jane Wallace. She and my mother traveled together and became very good friends. When they would come to St. Louis, to the Masonic Cathedral on Olive, they stayed at the Melbourne Hotel, only half a block from the cathedral. I always made it a point to go to the Melbourne to comb their hair for the Eastern Star's very formal parties. I also met President Truman's vice president, Alben Barkley. When he was married in the Methodist Church on Kingshighway, I did his bride's hair.

Rose Kennedy, mother of President John Kennedy, came to St. Louis twice that I can remember. She and her daughter Rosemary came for the Rose Ball, a fundraiser. Mrs. Kennedy's Washington hairstylist suggested that she see me when she was in St. Louis. She was perfectly charming. We styled Mrs. Kennedy's hair, and later I went to the ball.

I remember shaking President Johnson's hand when he stayed at the Chase Park Plaza. I swear it was the biggest hand I have ever shaken. It was *big*. And at an NHCA convention in Washington D.C., I met President and Mrs. Nixon. As National Styles Director of the NHCA that year, I escorted Mrs. Pat Nixon to the convention's fashion luncheon and also designed the "Pat-Tress" hairstyle, in her honor. The "Pat-Tress" was very casual, rather short. Flattering to the face.

During the Watergate era, I received a call from Washington asking me to do Martha Mitchell's hair. I was hesitant, but I agreed. After all, any publicity is good publicity. I was suggested to Mrs. Mitchell by Robin Weir, one of my friends in Washington, who was a hairdresser for Mrs. Reagan. The controversial Mrs. Mitchell arrived in St. Louis accompanied by several bodyguards and *Life Magazine* photographers. In spite of all I had heard about her and about how she spoke her mind, she was perfectly delightful. And the photos were in practically every big newspaper in the United States, in addition to *Life Magazine*.

In 1984, the NHCA named Betty Ford "Style Maker of the Year." She was scheduled to attend our convention in Las Vegas but was ill. President Ford appeared in her place. He spent several days with us in Las Vegas and gave us a great address, but we still missed his wife. While attending an NHCA convention in Atlanta, Georgia, I met Maureen Reagan and President George H.W. Bush.

I was privileged to wait on Mrs. Winthrop Rockefeller on several occasions. One particular instance stands out in my mind. I was with Mrs. Rockefeller, in her suite at the Park Plaza, for breakfast and to do her hair before she left to promote her book at one of our leading department stores, Stix Baer & Fuller. When Governor Rockefeller called to tell his wife of the birth of their first grandchild, I answered the phone and relayed the welcome message to Mrs. Rockefeller.

Demanding, but enjoyable, Princess Marcella Borghese of Italy was in St. Louis promoting her Borghese Cosmetics line to downtown stores. She insisted that I work her in one morning, and I just couldn't do it. I was too busy. Instead, I went in early for her the next morning, at eight o'clock. She didn't show up. I was angry and a little hurt. Her business manager came down to apologize and wanted me to take her later in the day, but I refused to do so. Finally, her business manager said, "I really don't blame you, but please take her this time." I agreed, under one condition: She was to pay for the appointment she didn't keep as well as for the new appointment. She came on time. I did her hair on several occasions after that and always enjoyed her. The Princess invited me to the Borghese Palace in Rome, but I never had time to go.

Internationally esteemed Edna Emme was my mentor and friend. She was well known in the beauty industry as president of Godefroy Cosmetics and manufacturer of TRESemmé hair products, now owned by Alberto Culver. Miss Emme lived next door to me on Lindell Boulevard and often entertained relatives from Germany. When the visits occurred during the summer, I offered her guests the use of my swimming pool and came to serve Miss Emme's young niece, Silvia. Little did I or anyone else know that the King of Sweden would fall in love with Silvia years later, when she served as an interpreter at the Olympic Games in Vienna. I was invited to the wedding but had to decline.

Queen Silvia's mother later said she had to pinch herself as she enjoyed lunch with her daughter at a sidewalk café in Sweden. As people passed by, they would pause to curtsey to the Queen—her daughter. It was like a fairytale.

Miss Emme once had so many houseguests that she made arrangements for Silvia, a teenager at the time, to stay at the Chase Park Plaza. But Silvia did not like the plan. "We don't have an extra bed," Miss Emme explained. "The only extra bed we have is in Uda's room." Uda was Miss Emme's housekeeper.

"I'd much rather sleep in Uda's room," Silvia stated. And so she did.

Sometime after Silvia's marriage to the King, Uda said, "Buddy, I'm the only person I know who ever slept with a real queen."

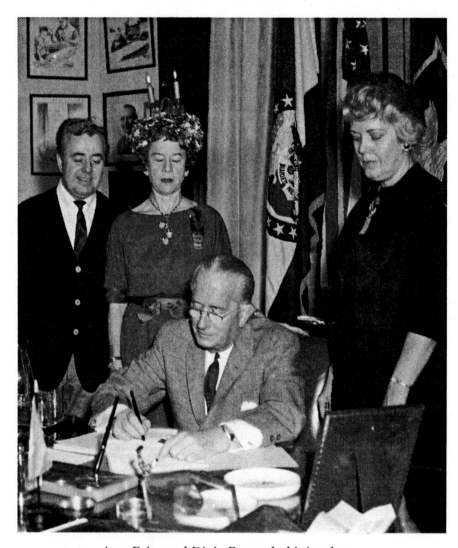

Ann Pritz and Dixie Rosenthal joined me,
as Mayor Tucker of St. Louis signed a proclamation for
National Beauty Salon Week.
Photo by ABK Photo Service

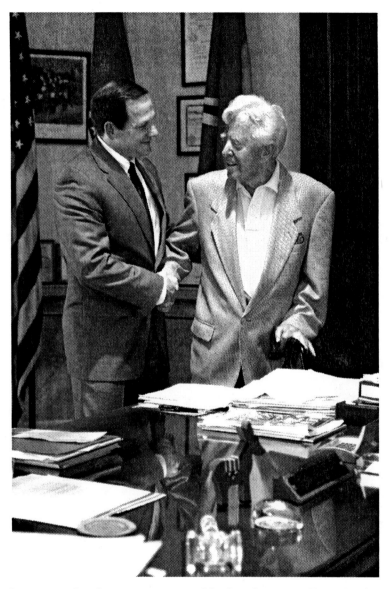

I am proud to be a supporter of St. Louis mayor Francis Slay.
Photo by Durb Curlee

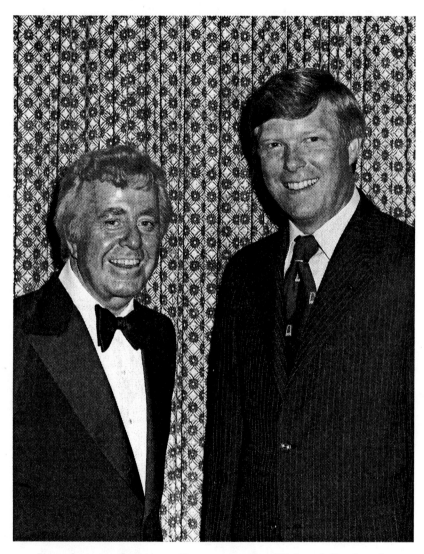

I was honored to meet Representative Richard Gephardt
when he appeared as guest speaker for a St. Louis Hair
Association meeting at the Steeplechase Club.
Photo by Robert Eichhorn—Eye to Eye Photography

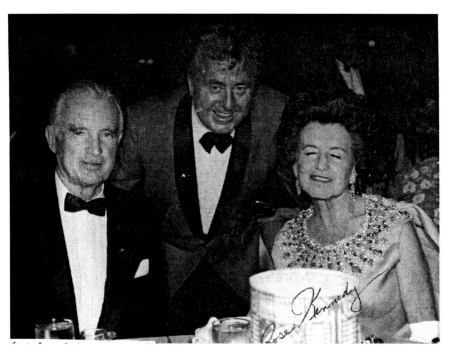

Rose Kennedy dined with U.S. Senator Stuart Symington at the Rose Ball, a St. Louis fundraiser.

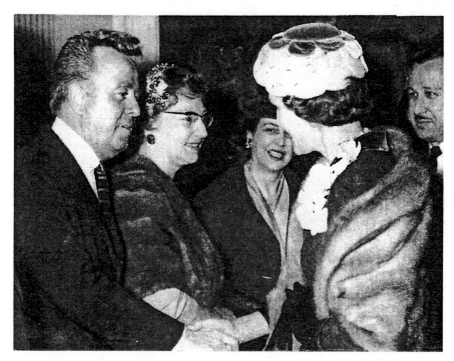

I not only met Mrs. Pat Nixon, I escorted her to the NHCA
convention luncheon in Washington D.C., at which I served
as chairman. Also pictured are, left to right, Evelyn Bunge,
Edna Emme, and Florian Harvat.

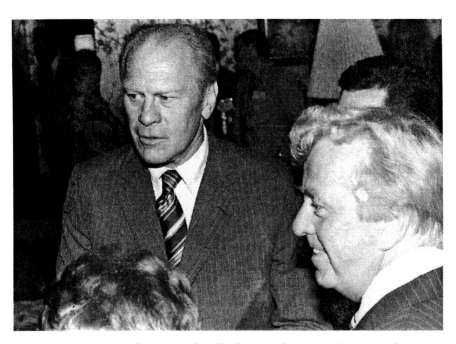

President Ford graciously filled in for his wife, Betty, at the 1984 NHCA convention in Las Vegas. Mrs. Ford, who was unable to attend due to illness, had been named NHCA's "Style Maker of the Year."

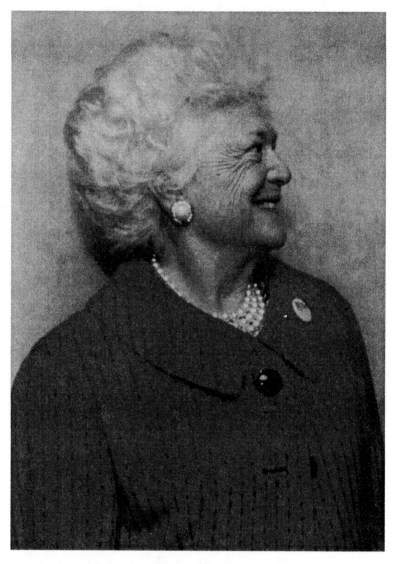

This photo of Barbara Bush was taken after Ron Coleman, one of my stylists, did her hair. Mrs. Bush was in St. Louis with her husband, who was taking part in a presidential debate.

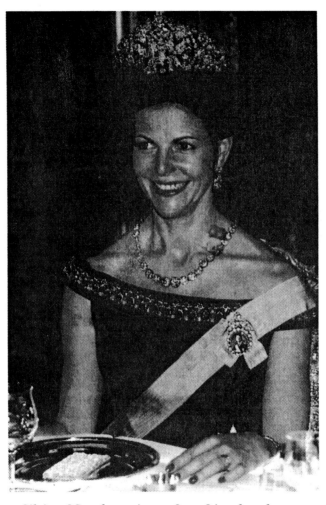

Queen Silvia of Sweden, niece of my friend and mentor, Miss
Edna Emme, was beautiful even before she was a queen. She
and the King have three children.

Look Who's Here

Celebrities came to St. Louis for all sorts of reasons, and most of them stayed at the Chase Park Plaza Hotel. Many were referred to me by their home hairdressers, who were friends of mine through my participation in the NHCA. Others were referred to me by my St. Louis customers. I was once preparing Mrs. Betty Grossman for styling when she asked, "Buddy, would you do me a favor?"

I said, "You know I will if I can, Mrs. Grossman." She was such a wonderful person and a fine client.

"I have a friend who is begging me to get her an appointment with you. Can you do her on Saturday?"

I checked my books and found that the only time I had was at eight o'clock in the morning, which she said was far too early for her friend, who worked until late at night. After much discussion, Mrs. Grossman divulged the name of her friend—Margo Fontaine, the great ballet dancer, who was dancing at the Muny, St. Louis' historical outdoor musical theater. I had no choice but to come in early, even for Miss Fontaine. Mrs. Grossman called Miss Fontaine and learned that she was willing. The great Dame Margo Fontaine! To think that she would get up early for me! She had her hair colored and styled for the ballet that evening.

Miss Fontaine's dance partner, Nureyev, once asked me to trim his hair. Another time, he fell on the street by the Plaza and scratched his face. He came up to the salon, and we applied some makeup to cover the mark. He danced very beautifully that evening, as usual. They were in town several times and always made it a point to come and see me.

Jane Pauley, who grew up in nearby Indiana, once arrived at the Chase Park Plaza to meet eight or ten of her former schoolmates, and I was asked to do her hair. When she arrived, I was quite surprised to find that she was wearing her hair in a French braid. Believe it or not, I do not French braid. I remembered I had a young man at my Plaza Frontenac salon, Louie, who did and brought him in by cab to do Jane Pauley's hair. That was embarrassing enough, but Jerry Berger made note of it in his gossip column. It wasn't the type of publicity I liked, but I did laugh about it. After all, it was true.

Abigail van Buren, well known for her "Dear Abby" column that has appeared for decades in many newspapers throughout the United States, was a salon regular when she stayed at the Chase Park Plaza. She's brilliant—she made it big on her own, which I admire. As she was leaving the salon one day, I said to her, "Do you mind, would you have some remembrance that I could keep?" She said she would and soon returned to the salon with a signed copy of one of her books. Inside the cover she had written, "Dear Buddy, You go to my head! Abigail."

Through the years, I had the honor of serving some of the most beautiful women in the world. Many of St. Louis' Veiled Prophet Queens were clients of mine, including Ann Desloge Werner, Carol Moon Gardner, Trudy Busch, Laura Rand Orthwein, and her daughter, Laura Orthwein. When the Miss America Pageant and the Miss Universe Pageant were held in St. Louis, on separate occasions, I was one of the hairdressers asked by the St. Louis Chamber of Commerce to be responsible for some of the contestants' hair. Miss New Zealand was crowned Miss Universe, but I was not fortunate enough to have done her hair; my friend and competitor Preston did her hair. I was also once honored to meet the first Jewish Miss America, Bess Myerson, crowned in 1945.

I had only been at the Chase Park Plaza a short time when I was called to do flamboyant wrestler Gorgeous George's hair. He approached through the hotel lobby, to the elevators, and into my salon in his traditional cloud of disinfectant and perfume, and surrounded by television cameras.

Gorgeous George, who wore his hair long, wavy, and bleached blond as part of his outrageous image, needed color. It just so happened that I was doing Carol Channing's hair at the same time. Later, during her show at the Chase Club, Miss Channing joked that her hairdresser, Buddy Walton, may have overbleached her hair because he was more interested in doing Gorgeous George's color than hers. I wouldn't do that, of course, especially not to Carol Channing.

Gorgeous George was picked up from my salon and taken to the Arena, St. Louis' largest exhibition building, for his match. He always invited me to his matches, and I went several times. The fans around me would call Gorgeous George names and shout out about his gold Georgie pins, which were gold-colored bobby pins that he wore in his long hair and threw into the audience during the match. I always wore a Georgie pin at Gorgeous George's matches and kept them for souvenirs.

Years later, the Shenkers inivited me to their daughter Patty's wedding in Vegas at the Dunes Hotel, which they owned. The wedding party lasted for three days. At the beautiful reception for over a thousand people, I met many celebrities, including Muhammad Ali. He was friendly and very funny. When he learned that I was a hairdresser, he reached out and started to gently twist a strand of my hair around his finger. I said, "Muhammad, if you do that I'm going to have to knock you on your…"

As big as he was, and in spite of who he was, he had to laugh. "Yes, Buddy, I'm sure you would."

While in Las Vegas, I did Patty's hair for her wedding. I also did Mrs. Shenker's hair, and some of the relatives' hair. It was a great time in my life. I had a magnificent suite and was treated like a king, like family, all expenses paid. Mrs. Shenker and her parents, the Koplars, contributed so much to my life. When Mrs. Shenker died, I was a pallbearer.

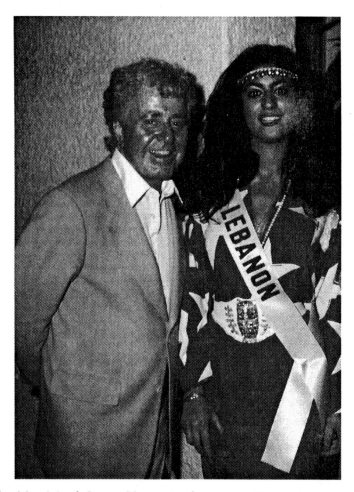

The Municipal Opera House in downtown St. Louis was once the site of the Miss Universe Pageant. I enjoyed helping many of the contestants with their hair.

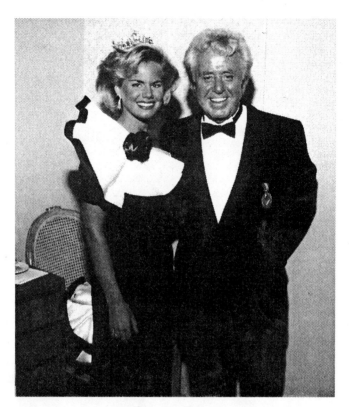

This is Miss America 1988. I was invited to many of the Miss
America Pageants.

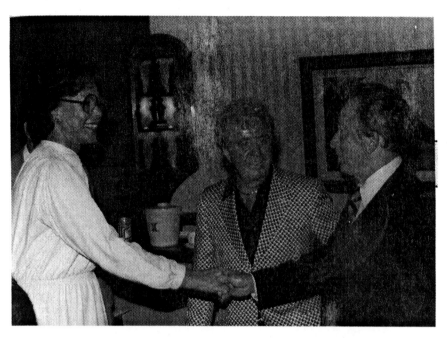

I was honored to meet one of the most well-known former
Miss Americas, Bess Myerson, who did much to promote
racial tolerance. Florian Harvat, past president of the NHCA,
is shaking her hand.

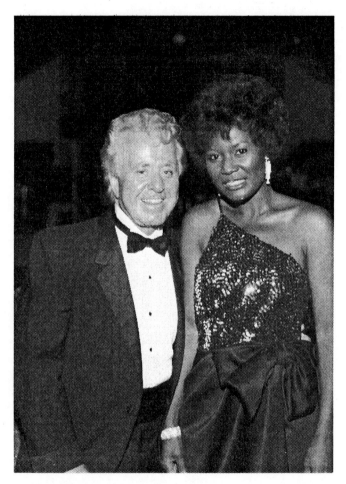

I served as a judge for the Mrs. America Pageant in 1984. I
believe that the winner, Brenda Williams, was the first black
Mrs. America.

Photo by Pro-Image, Ltd., Minneapolis, Minnesota

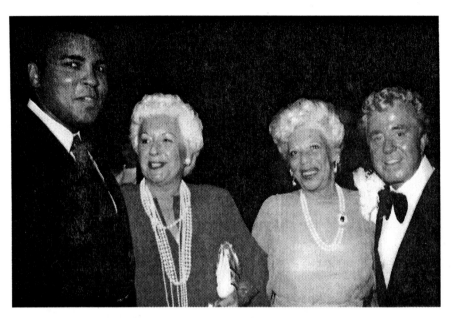

Muhammad Ali was only one of the celebrities I met when the Shenkers, owners of the Dunes Hotel, flew me to Las Vegas for their daughter Patty's wedding. Mrs. Shenker is standing next to me in this photo. At her side is Tody Barnett, her cousin.

Shaping the Stars

Working in the Chase Park Plaza, where all the stars stayed when they were in town, I met many famous performers, such as Ruby Keeler, Rosemary Clooney, and Phyllis Diller. Miss Marjorie Main came in for a facial and makeup and lost a five-carat diamond ring. The police found it on the floor in the facial room. Joan Bennett was in St. Louis for a charity event and had her hair done. Very simple, very plain. She was a very pretty woman. Bette Davis was in once—lovely lady. Everyone wanted to see her; everyone wanted to talk to her. The commotion could have driven her wild, but she was nice to everyone. Rosemary Clooney was appearing at the Chase Club. After I styled her hair, she invited Ron Coleman, one of my hairdressers, and me to dinner in the Tenderloin Room, in the Chase Park Plaza. She was a beautiful lady.

Oscar-winning actress Joan Crawford was another beautiful lady. I have admired Joan Crawford all my life and will always remember her visit to my salon. When I was asked to do her hair, they sent me her itinerary. Even the president of the United States doesn't have an itinerary like hers. Every thirty minutes of the day she was to be at a certain place: 10:00 a.m.—Arrive at Buddy Walton's Salon. 10:30—Pepsi Cola to be served—she was on Pepsi's board of directors at that time and relentlessly promoted the drink, even in her movies. 11:00—Hair to be combed by hair-dresser Buddy Walton. Her day was filled.

Broadway star Beatrice Lilly stayed at the Chase Park Plaza Hotel when she was performing in town, and I had the privilege of doing her hair. I called a friend of mine, a hairstylist in Chicago, to tell him that I was doing Bea Lilly's hair. He said, "Buddy, I have to tell you something about doing Bea Lilly's hair. You know she was a titled lady of England. She was called Lady Peel. A friend of mine was doing Lady Peel's hair and was running over on the time. His next client, Mrs. Swift, kept making a fuss to the receptionist about him being late for her appointment. And Bea Lilly knew it. He was fifteen or twenty minutes late. When Miss Lilly came out, she went to the desk and said to the recep-tionist, 'Would you mind telling Mrs. Swift, the butcher's wife, that Lady Peel is finished?'"

Tallulah Bankhead, scandalous star of stage, screen, television, and radio, was unforgettable. I had read in some magazine that she didn't wear any underclothes. Well, someone in California recommended that she call me to do her hair when she was in St. Louis. I was sitting at my desk, and when I looked up, coming across the mezzanine toward the salon was Tallulah Bankhead, actresses Polly Bergen and Billie Burke, and a handsome young man carrying a little white poodle. They were almost marching. It looked like a parade.

"Miss Bankhead," I said when she arrived at the salon, "would you prefer a private booth, or would you like me to style your hair at one of the open stations?"

"Oh, no. No, *dahling*. I want a private booth."

I asked my porter, Clinton, to take her to a private booth. When I came in, I said, "Miss Bankhead, would you like coffee?"

"Oh, yes, *dahling*. Lots and lots of black coffee."

I asked Clinton to bring her a pot of black coffee. She took a drink and immediately spit it out onto the wall. She said, "When I order coffee, I want *hot* coffee, not warm p_ _ _!"

It made me so angry I didn't know what to do. I called Clinton to clean up the mess that she had made in her booth, and he did. Politely, I asked, "Miss Bankhead, do you prefer a smock or do you want to leave your dress on?"

"I'd like a smock, *dahling*," she said. I gave her a smock and left the booth, so she could change. When I returned to the booth, I quickly saw that what I had read was true. Miss Bankhead, lying back in the shampoo chair, had neglected to button up the smock. She had on nothing underneath. I quickly walked out of the booth and asked my porter, Clinton, to go back in. I told him he needed to "clean up another mess." When he entered the booth and saw what I had seen, he was so embarrassed he almost fainted. It was wrong of me to send Clinton in; I apologized to him. But in the end, I did enjoy doing Miss Bankhead's hair very much.

Bob Hope's wife, Dolores, was an enjoyable client. She had her hair shampooed and styled in my salon more than once. Their daughters, in school at St. Louis University, were also in the salon several times. Bob always came in to say hello. Sometimes he would stay to joke with us for half an hour or so, and the ladies were always thrilled to see him. He was a funny man, constantly funny.

I spent more time with actress Kathy Crosby, wife of Bing Crosby, than with any other actress. A movie was being made in St. Louis—*The Hoodlum Priest,* sort of a gangster or hoodlum picture, starring Kathy Crosby and Don Murray. Of course, it also had many St. Louis people in it. They shot a lot of it at Alma and Harry Kessler's home and at area country clubs. I was the top stylist and spent every day for several months with the cast and crew. From scene to scene, a week later or a day later, I had to be careful to copy the styles that I had done earlier in the movie. On the weekends, Bing would come to town. I had lunch or dinner with him several times, and between his visits I spent a lot of evenings going out for dinner with Kathy and her mother, who was with her. I had top billing as hairdresser in the credits of the movie. I saw the movie a couple of times. It was good. But not too good.

I was *friendly* with Kathy Crosby, but Martha Raye was a true *friend.* I can't say enough about her. I did her hair many, many times. We met in Florida, where she owned a cocktail lounge. We went to cocktail parties together in Florida and in St. Louis. She came to my home, and she loved to cook—I have a picture of her that was taken while she was cooking in my kitchen. She made some sort of a goulash; I think it was Hungarian Goulash. Martha Raye was one of my great friends for years. My friend Sam was crazy about her. She was the tops.

Vaudeville entertainer Sophie Tucker was a friend, too, and the Last of the Red Hot Mamas. She might be in California; she might be in New York; she might be in Europe. But when she was making plans to be in St. Louis, she called me for an appointment. I remember one time she called, and my receptionist said I couldn't come to the phone, not realizing it was Sophie Tucker. When I did get to the phone, I heard about it.

If I take the time to call you, you son of a b _ _ _ _, you'd better take the time to talk to me."

But I don't blame her, because that was just Sophie. I did like her very much, and she was always great to me. She once had a party at the Chase Club for my mother and father. That's the type of lady she was.

Often, I would sit with her at her book signings. So many of her fans pestered her, saying, in their syrupy voices, things like, "Sophie, remember me? I met you when Mrs. De Schutz gave a party for you in L.A and…"

Sophie would interrupt. "G_ _ d_ _ _ _ _, I can't remember all of you. I've met a lot of people. Either get a book or get out of line."

I would say to her, "Sophie, if I were that lady, I would never buy your book."

But she said, "They know I don't mean it."

Sophie pulled her hair away from her face because she perspired a lot. In fact, as she sang and danced on the stage, she used a long kerchief to blot the perspiration from her face. She appeared to have long hair, but her hair was actually cut very short in the back, from ear to ear. From the top of her head down, the hair was ten to twelve inches long. I used to put it up in a French roll. I'd pull it up to the front and give her height. She had beautiful, beautiful hair, and she was a beautiful lady. And a character.

Another character who frequented the shop was Phyllis Diller— she really is as wacky as she seems on television. The reception area in my salon was quite large. Women would be waiting there for their hairdresser, and Phyllis would come in. And instead of walking, she would *sashay* in. She'd look around with that expression on her face that we all know, and she'd say, "Well, come on, ladies, brighten up! We're going to have an orgy!" You never knew what would come out of that lady's mouth.

Phyllis had a home in Kirkwood, Missouri, and her daughters also frequented my salon. I did Phyllis' wigs, mostly. They were always sort of "fright" wigs. I did color her hair a little, but I never had to worry too much about her hair—she almost always had on a turban. Or I would do her hair, and then she would put on a wig.

The salon also came alive when any of the sexy Gabor sisters came in. In fact, it would jump with excitement. They were all lively and friendly; they were glamorous, beautiful women who dressed beautifully. Everyone wanted to see them and to meet them—they were top stars and so popular at the time—and they were nice to everyone. Ava, Zsa Zsa, and Jolie, their mother, all had their hair lightened. Magda did not. They were always with Mrs. Alma Kessler, who was a very popular lady in town. Mrs. Kessler had a home in Palm Springs, and that is where the Gabors lived, I am told. For a long time, Magda lived in St. Louis, at the Park Plaza.

So many great performers came to St. Louis. Liberace came to town several times, and, as everyone knows, Liberace had poodles. He always called my friend Sam, at the Poodle Palace, to have his dogs groomed. He and Sam became friends, and he invited Sam and me to his show in Vegas. When we were there, people mistook Sam for Liberace and asked for his autograph. We enjoyed it very much. Helene Baskowitz, a client of mine and a friend, was often seen with Liberace when he was in town, playing in the Georgian Room of the hotel.

The names Martha Graham and Ethel Merman are forever connected in my memory. Both women, while staying at the Chase Park Plaza Hotel, told me they didn't think they should have to pay their bills. They believed that the honor of doing their hair should have been adequate pay. Of all the well-known people I've waited on, I've never had another person say that to me—just those two women, at different times. I told them both that I enjoyed doing their hair and did not need the publicity, and that if they ever came back in town I'd be happy to serve them again. I was nice to them. And they were very nice ladies, really.

Fashionable Rosalind Russell was one of America's great stars of stage and screen. I'll never forget what she said to me when I was styling her hair. "Buddy," she said, "you're a great hairdresser and a great person. I'd love for you to visit me sometime in California."

I considered that a great compliment, and I said, "Miss Russell, I doubt if I'll be in California, but thank you. If I ever do get out there, we could plan it when your hairdresser comes to your home to do your hair, and I could pick up a few points."

And she said, "Oh, Buddy, but you could teach him a lot. I wish you would come out."

Buddy Walton's Chase Park Plaza Salon. There'll never be another salon like it.

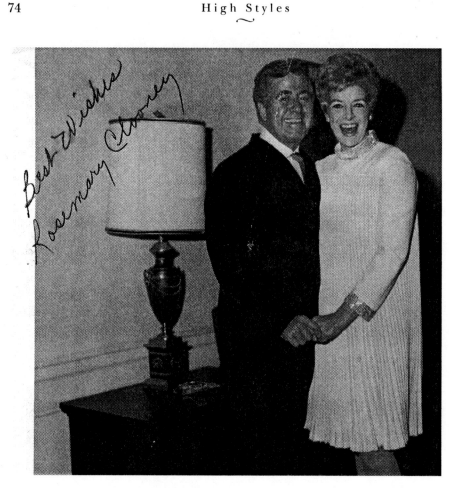

Rosemary Clooney and I were photographed in the Georgian
Room at the Park Plaza.

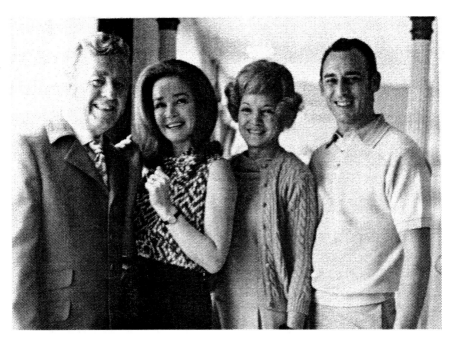

Kathy Crosby and I spent many hours together during the
filming of her movie. Marie, my receptionist, and Robert
Joehle, a talented hairdresser in my salon, enjoyed getting to
know Kathy, too.

Photo by Pictorial Press Service, St. Louis, Missouri

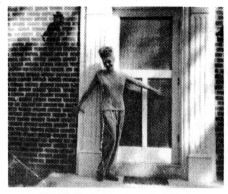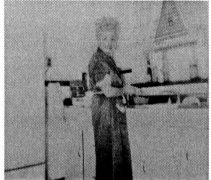

Martha Raye was a true friend. Here, in front of my house on
Lindell Boulevard, she saw my camera and quickly struck a
pose. Inside, Martha was cooking up something good in my
kitchen. She was so beautiful, her hair piled high on her head
like women did in those years.

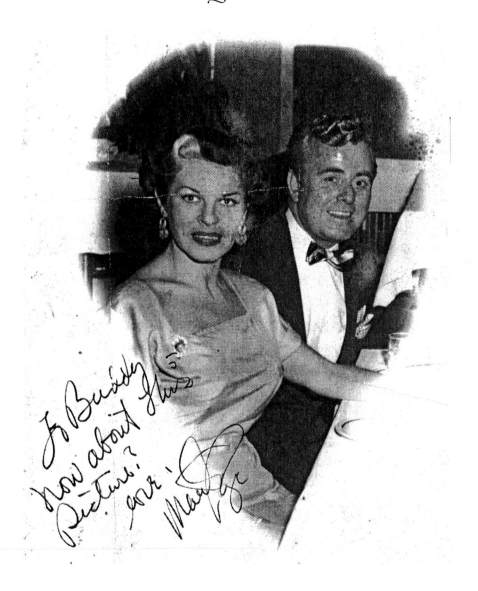

Martha Raye and I enjoyed getting "dressed" to go out on a
Friday or Saturday night. We remained friends for years.

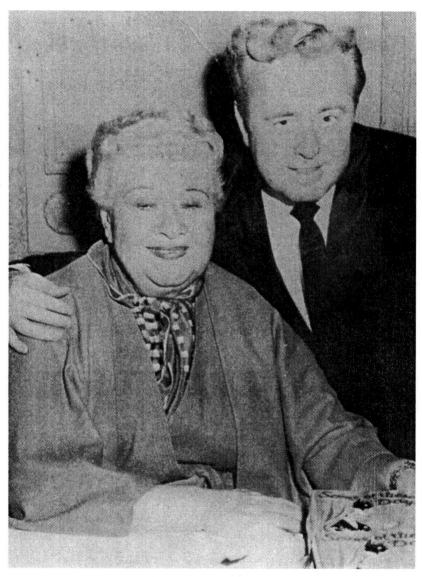

Sophie Tucker, "The Last of the Red Hot Mamas," was
another true friend.

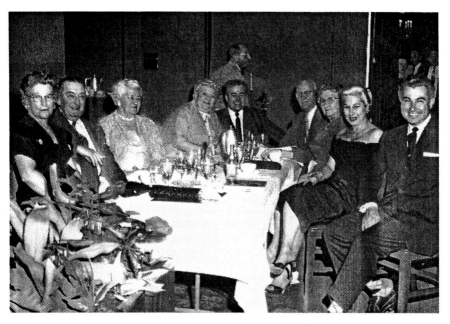

Sophie Tucker was a generous friend, as well. Sophie, on my
right hand side, threw this dinner party at the Chase Park
Plaza for my parents, who are seated to my left. My friend
Sam is on the far right of the photo.

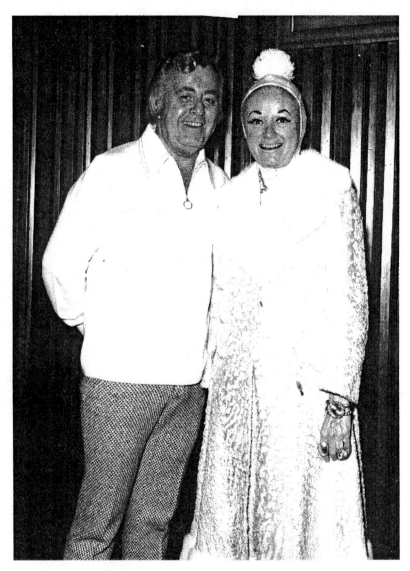

Phyllis Diller rarely appeared in public without a wig or a turban
over her hair. She once gave me a photo she had signed,
"Dearest Buddy—You flipped my wig!! Love, Phyllis Diller."

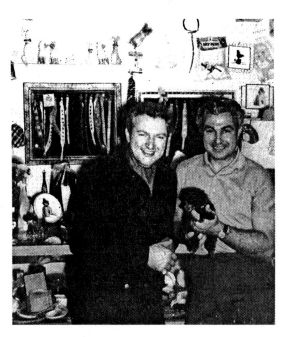

Liberace, on the left, and my friend Sam, on the right, really
do look a lot alike.

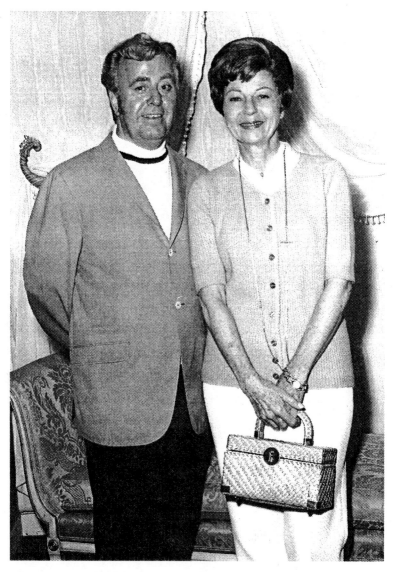

Perfect TV mom Harriett Nelson, of *The Adventures of Ozzie and Harriett,* posed for this photo in my salon after receiving our services.

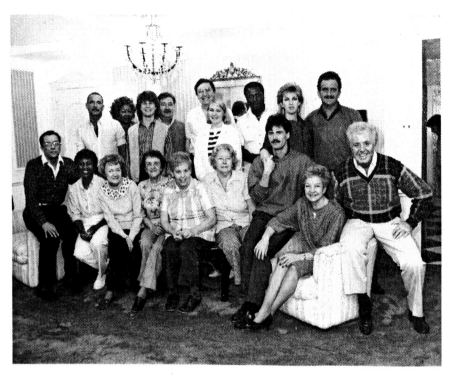

The world's greatest salon staff gathered for a photo at the
Chase Park Plaza. It could not have happened anywhere else.
After all, "The Chase is the Place."

Sitting Pretty

Shop Talk

My longtime bookkeeper at the Chase Park Plaza salon, Marge Graham, eventually moved to Florida, where she worked for the mayor of Fort Lauderdale. Through her, I was invited to open the first beauty salon on the Galt Ocean Mile, which was just then being developed. At that time, it was a strip of beautiful beach over a mile long, completely barren. Now it's all hotels.

Buddy Walton's Galt Ocean Mile Salon was a success. I later opened Pier 66 Beauty Salon, just north of the Galt Ocean Mile. Then came Lauderdale by the Sea Salon and, finally, Ocean Manor Salon. They all proved very successful. My friends Louella and Porter Bailey, of Duluth, Minnesota, later moved to Florida and bought half interest in my four salons. For many years, I spent the winters in my Florida apartment and came back to St. Louis for the spring and summer business.

When the beautiful Plaza Frontenac was being built in a suburb of St. Louis—Saks Fifth Avenue, Neiman Marcus, and all the top stores of St. Louis and beyond—I was contacted to open a salon. Space was terribly expensive, and I was frightened to do so. One of my clients who was a knowledgeable realtor, Miss Blanche Grossman, encouraged me. She convinced me that everything was moving west. In the end, as much as I hated to leave the Chase Park Plaza, I felt I had to move with the times. The top hairdressers and other professionals who worked with me helped me make Buddy Walton's Salon of Cosmetology another success story. I operated in Plaza Frontenac for nearly ten years before retiring and selling the salon to a hairdresser by the name of Sal Vitale. It has been sold several times since then and, at this writing, is known as the Green Door Day Spa.

One of the happiest moments in my career came in the form of another phone call from the Koplar family. Harold Koplar had taken over his father's position at the Chase Park Plaza. "Buddy, I'm going to be like Mom," he said. "Would you like to come home?" It seems the chain that had bought my salon at the Chase Park Plaza when I left hadn't been as successful as they expected to be. He gave the salon to me again. Again I went "back home" to the Chase Park Plaza, this time only briefly, as the hotel was later sold.

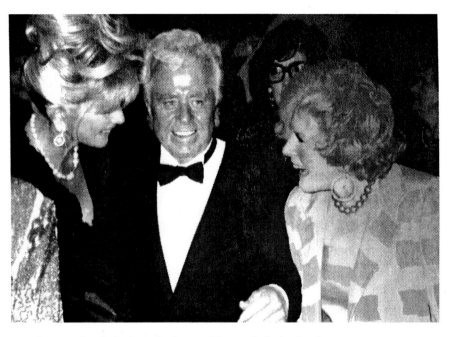

I was scheduled to do Ivana Trump's hair for her appearance
at the grand opening of one of the Plaza Frontenac
department stores, but she had to cancel at the last minute. I
attended the opening as a guest of Charlotte Cohen. Ivana's
hair was beautiful—it was long and blond, and she had pulled
it up casually.

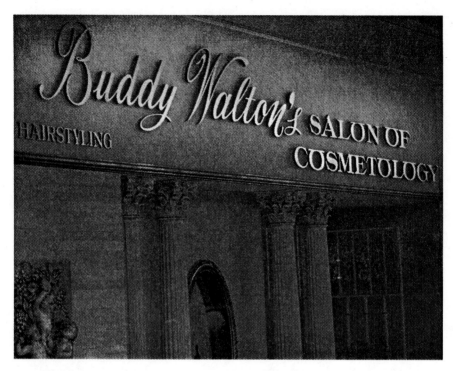

My Plaza Frontenac salon was one of three salons I owned in
St. Louis. I also owned four salons in Florida.

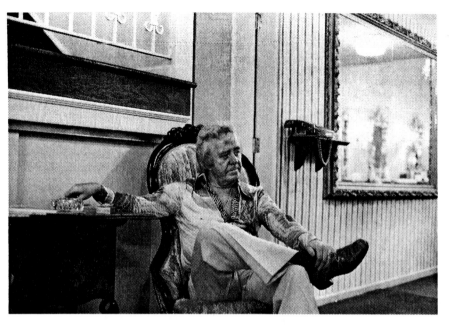

Here I am, taking a brief smoke break at my
Plaza Frontenac salon.

Highlights

I wanted to be the best. Maybe I *wasn't* the best, but I was *doing* my best. Generally, I didn't feel I was in competition with anyone in my work, though there were a couple of hairdressers in St. Louis who I wanted to stay above. They had both worked for me and then had gone out on their own, forming the Jon' Tomas salons, which became very successful serving a client base similar to mine. I don't know how they felt, but I didn't have any hard feelings. I was proud of their success, believing that I had given them a good start. So many young hairdressers came through my salons. One St. Louis salon owner told me, "I think everyone in St. Louis has worked for you, Buddy. Whenever we have an applicant, they write, 'Worked for Buddy Walton.'"

At one point, with my St. Louis and Florida shops combined, I employed approximately 150 people. When I interviewed someone for a position in my salons, there were two things I looked for. First, the person had to make you laugh while also being serious about work. Second, the person's appearance had to be clean and neat. I was busy. There was no way I could change a hairdresser's personality, and there was no way I could change a hairdresser's personal appearance. But I could make a dedicated hairdresser into a *good* hairdresser.

A good hairdresser has to consider a hairstyle in relation to the person who will be wearing it. No matter how great the style is, it has to fit the person. But the most important consideration is to please the customer. After I retired, a woman stopped me at the YWCA gym and said, "I hear you're a famous hairstylist. They tell me you've done such famous people—name some."

So I told her, "I've done several of the presidents' wives, including Mrs. Nixon…"

"Oh, well—I never liked her hair anyway," the woman said.

I couldn't let that pass. I said, "You know, I don't think she would have liked your hairstyle either." We laughed. The point is, please the customer.

My years as a hairdresser had ups and downs, but I had a very interesting life. Oh, there were times when it was boring, too, but it was good. Very good. I wouldn't mind doing it over again. One area of my career that contributed very much to my success, as well as to my enjoyment, was my involvement in professional organizations, specifically HairAmerica and the NHCA—the National Hairdresser and Cosmetologist Association.

I became a member of HairAmerica in 1955 and have served as both its chairman and its styles director. I served as director and as one of the trainers for the NHCA's first World Olympics of Hairdressing team, which competed in Paris in 1962. This is one of the highest honors in my profession. We spent five weeks in Europe and came in twelfth in the world, with thirty countries competing. I am honored that I was invited to serve as the United States representative to the Organization Artistic International, or OAI. I served for several years.

I have received the NHCA's prestigious Charles Award, and I was honored for my contributions and support of the international organization with the World Gold Medallion, its highest award, received by only five hairdressers in the United States. The other four recipients are Edna L. Emme, Marguerite Buck, Joseph Weir, and William Ware. This list of achievements sounds unbelievable, even to me, but it is completely true.

I attended all of the World Championships in which United States teams participated, as well as ten European Championships, representing the United States as a judge for ten of the events. I also served NHCA as chairman of the International Affairs Committee and served as advisor to the Canadian National Team at the World Championships in Tokyo, Japan. Truthfully, there was a time when I was frightened to do these things, but I thank God that I did.

After my many experiences as a competition judge, including the judging of World and European Championships, NHCA designated me as *Judge de Honeur*, which entitled me to judge in any contest arena, in Europe or the United States. I have also received the Edna L. Emme International Medallion and Lifetime Achievement Awards in St. Louis and in Missouri. I was one of the first five inductees into the NHCA Hall of Renown and was nominated to the Hairdressing Hall of Fame.

One honor of which I am particularly proud is my unanimous election to the Mine au Breton Historical Society "Gallery of Washington County Notables." The sixtieth person elected, I am in good company: Others elected include Stephen Austin, the Father of Texas; an Arkansas Supreme Court judge; a Missouri governor; a United States senator, and a Manhattan Project scientist.

I am honored to have my name on a number of trophies, within Missouri as well as nationwide, such as Buddy Walton's Roving Cup. Recently, I received notice that the International Buddy Walton Trophy and International Medallion will be presented annually at the new "BeautyFUSION NY" held in conjunction with the Health and Beauty America Show, one of the premier beauty events in the industry. The event will take place at the Jacob K. Javits Convention Center in New York City.

How could all this have happened? How could it have happened to *me*? I feel my life has been a gift. I have been blessed. I don't really know why or how it happened, but it seems that if you dream and believe in your dreams, if you do good work and try to do right by people, you can be successful at what you love. And for as long as I can remember, I have loved working with people's hair.

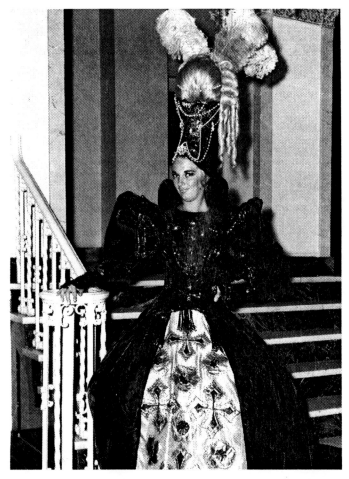

Robert Joehle, one of my talented hairdressers, worked with
me to present this Historical Fantasy Hairstyle at the 1961
Mississippi Valley Show, held at the Chase Park Plaza Hotel.
This work of art was inspired by similar styles presented at the
1960 World Championships in Paris and was the first Fantasy
Hairstyle created by a United States hairdresser. Model Carlene
Jones stood over nine and a half feet tall, including hair.
Photo by ABK Photo Service

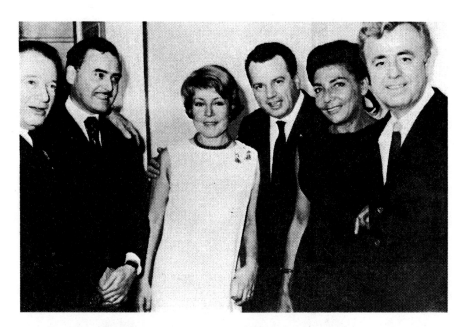

In Paris, in 1968, we were considered the six most renowned
hairdressers in the world. From left to right: Guillame, of
Paris; Alexandre, of Paris and Madrid; one Carita sister; Para,
hairdresser to the Queen of England; the second Carita sister;
and me. I was once in the room while Para combed the
Queen's hair—it was a thrill to be so near the
Queen of England.

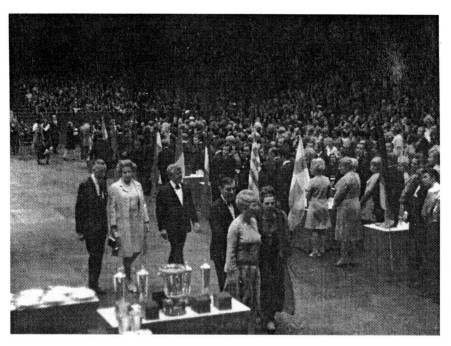

The World Olympics of Hairdressing award ceremony, held in
Germany in 1970, was exciting and moving. That's me, Judge
of Honor, front and center.

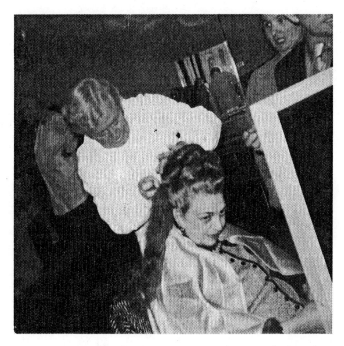

In Moscow, in 1972, Miss Emme was my model for the first
American hairdressing demonstration in Russia.

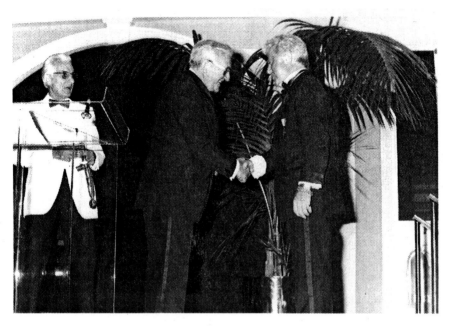

Pierre Masson, Secretary General of Coiffure International Congress (CIC) and one of the top hairdressers in Paris, looked on as President General Dr. Ferdinand Leibundgut awarded me the World Gold Medallion in Stuttgart, in 1974.

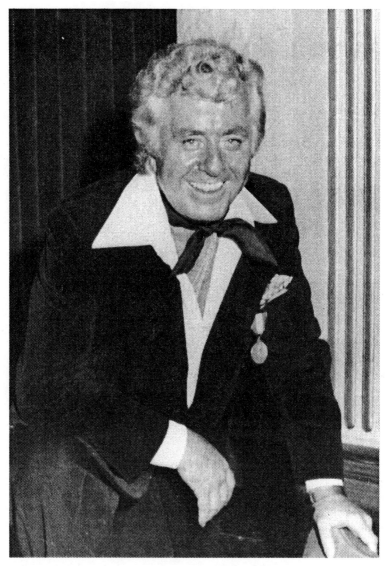

I was one of only five American hairdressers to receive the prestigious World Gold Medallion in recognition of my contributions to the beauty industry.

USA HAIRDRESSING TEAM DIRECTOR AND TRAINER

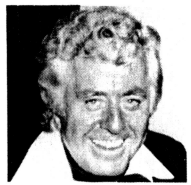

Team Director–Buddy Walton, St. Louis, MO

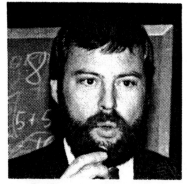

Team Trainer–Michael Taylor, Denver, CO

USA JUDGES FOR THE WORLD CHAMPIONSHIPS

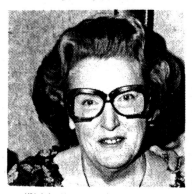

USA Judge–Marguerite Buck, New York, NY

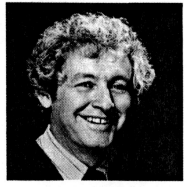

USA Judge–Leo Passage, Chicago, IL

The Board of Directors of the National Hairdressers and Cosmetologists Association has named Buddy Walton of St. Louis, MO, and Michael Taylor of Denver, CO, as Team Director and Trainer, respectively, for the 1980 USA Hairdressing Team which will be competing in the World Championships of Hairdressing to be held September 21–23 in Rotterdam, the Netherlands.

NHCA also announced that Marguerite Buck of New York, NY, and Leo Passage of Chicago, IL, will be representing the United States as judges at the World Championships.

This page appeared in the NHCA newsletter, announcing my appointment as Team Director of the 1980 USA Hairdressing Team, which competed in the World Championships of Hairdressing in Rotterdam, the Netherlands.

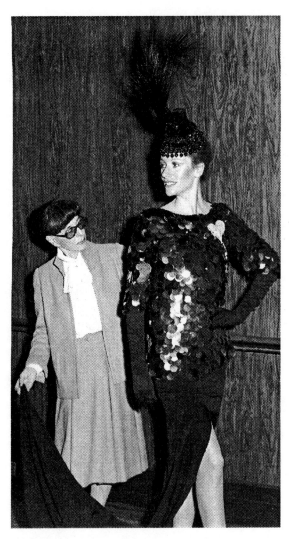

Edyth Head, Hollywood's most celebrated clothing designer, arranges her gown on a convention model in Las Vegas, in 1981. Alida Weergang, a top U.S. hairdresser, convinced Edyth Head to participate. It was unusual for her to agree to take part in anything other than movies.

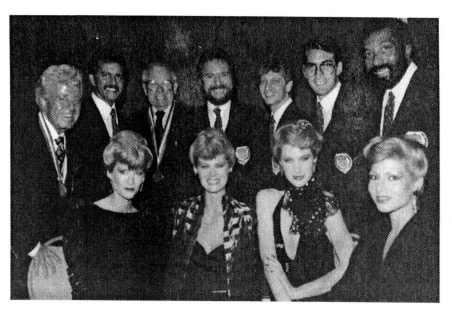

The 1982 United States Hair Olympic Team appears here
with our beautiful models. I served as captain of the team,
which competed in Holland.

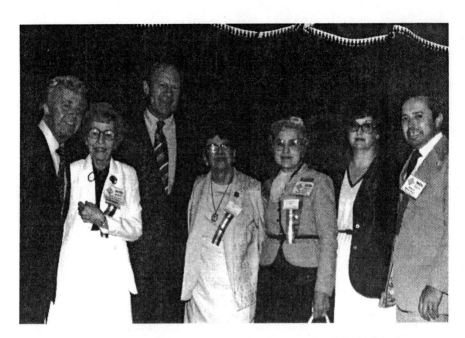

In addition to President Ford and yours truly, this 1984 photo
includes, left to right, NHCA past presidents Vanek, Emme,
and Aitken, followed by Mrs. Berger and her husband, Tom
Berger, my good friend.

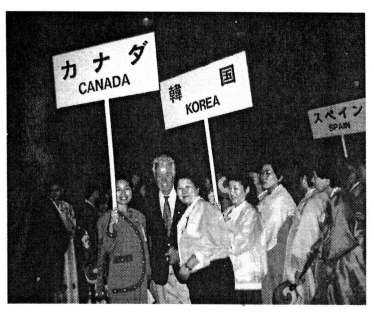

In 1992, I traveled to Tokyo, Japan as Team Advisor for
Canada's World Olympic Hairdressing Team.

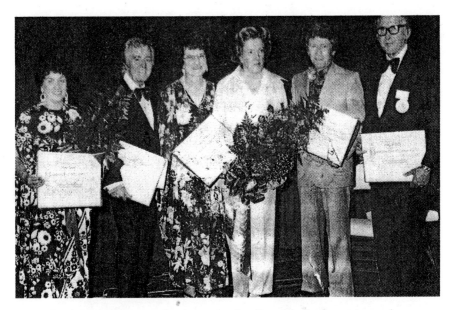

It was an honor to be among the first five inductees to the
National Cosmetology Association's Hairstyling Hall of
Renown. Left to right, those honored are from Minneapolis,
St. Louis (that's me, of course), Illinois (then-current
president of NHCA), New York (originally from Switzerland—
my good friend Marguerite Buck), New Jersey,
and Oklahoma.

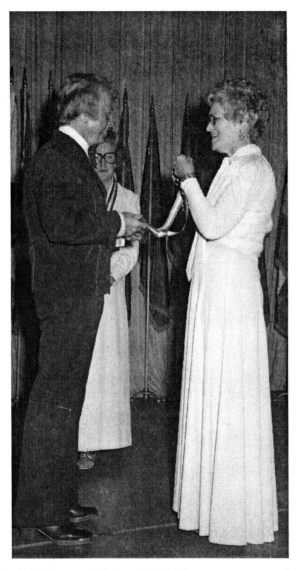

Jonnie McCoy, president of NHCA, presents me with the
Emme Medallion at a convention in Ocean City, Maryland, as
my friend Marguerite Buck looks on.

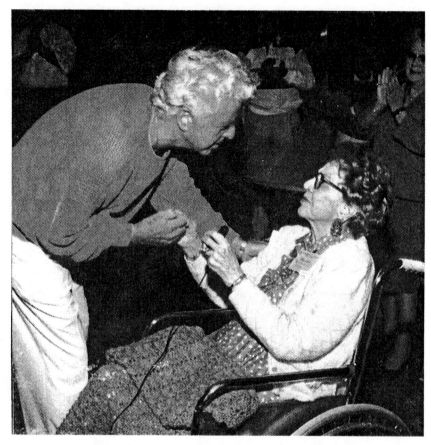

Dear Miss Emme greatly honored me at an NHCA convention when she presented me with the celebrated Mr. Godefroy's ring.

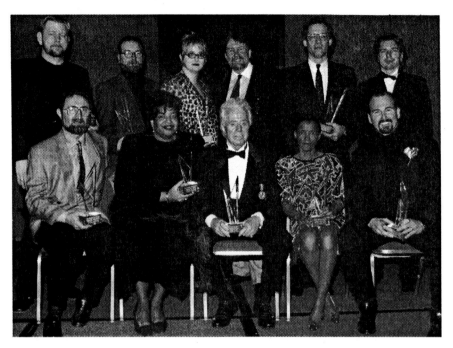

Local hairdressers paid me a great compliment. All of the hairdressers pictured received St. Louis Lifetime Achievement awards; I was honored with the top award.

About the Authors

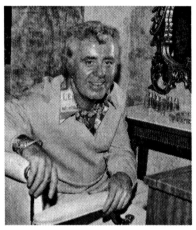

Buddy Walton found success doing what he always loved most—working with hair. A licensed cosmetologist for more than fifty-five years, he was awarded the National Hairdresser and Cosmetologist Association's World Gold Medallion, its highest honor. Now retired, Buddy lives in St. Louis, Missouri, where he thinks about hair every day.

Connie McIntyre helps people capture their stories in unique books. She has authored and created dozens of handcrafted keepsake books and several commercially bound books, and is coauthor of *Upside Downside Inside Out—Poems about Being a Kid*. Connie lives in St. Louis with her husband and their three very tall children.

0-595-31875-4

Printed in the United States
23761LVS00006B/148-153